The Most Pressing Health Issues of the Modern World

The Most Pressing Health Issues of the Modern World

Austin Mardon
Michael Tang
Rebecca Dang
Aida Zaheer
Lilian Yeung
Francis Fernandes

Edited by Catherine Mardon

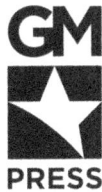

GM
★
PRESS

Cover Design & Typeset by Joshua Kramer

Print ISBN: 978-1-77369-830-4
eBook ISBN: 978-1-77369-831-1

Golden Meteorite Press
103 11919 82 St NW
Edmonton, AB T5B 2W3
www.goldenmeteoritepress.com

Contents

Chapter 1: An Introduction to Prominent Health Issues in 21st Century Canada
By Michael Tang

Similar to other developed nations, the most pressing health issues in Canada include noncommunicable, chronic diseases. Some prominent examples include diabetes, cardiovascular diseases (CVD), chronic respiratory diseases (CRD), and cancer. These 4 diseases are responsible for about two thirds of all deaths in Canada every year.[1] Overall, chronic conditions make up some of the leading causes of death in Canada and are preventable as there are modifiable risk factors that can be addressed.

Beyond mortality, other health conditions such as mood and anxiety disorders are significant causes of disability among Canadians and greatly contribute to healthcare expenditures. In fact, the four chronic diseases mentioned above and mood and anxiety disorders combine to account for around one third of direct healthcare expenditure in Canada.[2] There is also the possibility of multi-morbidity, where a person may experience physical, chronic conditions alongside conditions such as mood and anxiety disorders. This is relatively more common among the elderly population, which makes these conditions an especially pressing issue given Canada's aging population.[3] The impact of mental health conditions is also exacerbated by issues such as stigma and barriers to mental health care access, such as insufficient fundings for services, long wait times, high costs, and not knowing where to get help.[4]

Related to mental health is substance abuse, or the problematic use of psychoactive drugs such as alcohol, opioids, and cannabis.[5] The

1   Public Health Agency of Canada, 2017
2   Public Health Agency of Canada, 2017
3   Public Health Agency of Canada, 2017
4   Moroz et al., 2020
5   Health Canada, 2018

use of these psychoactive drugs in a certain manner, frequency, situation, or amount can potentially cause harm to individuals, their families/social networks, and the broader community.[6] These harmful impacts can include health issues and problematic behaviours such as drunk driving. Problematic use of substances is a serious issue in Canada, with an estimated 1 in 5 of Canadians aged 15 years or older experiencing a substance use disorder in their lifetime.[7] Some of the root causes or contributing factors behind problematic substance use include adverse childhood experiences, poor academic performance, and unemployment.[8] Most if not all of these causes/factors are difficult to address, which could explain why substance abuse remains a pressing health concern in Canada.

Canada's population, like many other high-income countries, is rapidly aging due to factors such as decreased birth rates and increases in life expectancy.[9] In 2017, nearly one sixth of Canada's population (5.8 million) was 65 years or older. The 65+ age group is expected to grow at around 4 times the rate of the overall population. This is one of the contributing factors behind the severity of chronic diseases as the risk of these diseases does increase to a certain extent as a person gets older, potentially due to the accumulation of exposures and risk factors over a lifetime.

Certain elements of the general modern lifestyle can also contribute to chronic diseases. First, the development of technology and transportation has led to a more sedentary lifestyle that does not exactly promote physical exercise. Motor vehicles and other forms of transportation have greatly increased the potential for travel and daily commute but have reduced the need for walking and other forms of transportation/travel involving physical exercise. Additionally, widespread uses of technology such as smartphones and computers has also contributed to a more sedentary lifestyle. Finally, the modern diet often features a significant amount of

---

6   Health Canada, 2018
7   Health Canada, 2018
8   Health Canada, 2018
9   Lee & Smith, 2018

processed foods, which are often high in sodium and fat. High sodium and fat consumption can contribute to cardiovascular conditions such as hypertension.

Given this context, it makes sense why Canada's most pressing health issues include chronic conditions, mental health conditions, and substance use. This book will focus on six of the key health issues affecting 21st century Canada: diabetes, cancer, CVDs, obesity, substance abuse (including the opioid crisis), and Parkinson's disease.

The Risk Factors and Conditions Behind These Pressing Health Issues

In general, there are several "determinants of health" that range from biological factors to unhealthy behaviours to socioeconomic factors. Of these determinants, there are 4 specific risk factors for chronic diseases and other health conditions that the large majority of Canadians have one or more of. Whether it be caused by the modern Western lifestyle, societal norms, or personal decisions, many Canadians display one or more of the following risk factors: smoking, physical inactivity, harmful use of alcohol, and unhealthy eating.[10]

First, tobacco smoking is linked to several chronic diseases, such as cancer, CVDs, and CRDs.[11] Tobacco products often contain ingredients that are toxic to several organ systems and generally have a negative impact on overall physical health. While smoking rates in Canada have been decreasing throughout the past few decades, smoking unfortunately remains the leading risk factor behind preventable deaths.[12] In 2014, around 17.9% (over 5 million) of Canadians aged 12 or older smoked on a daily or occasional basis. However, there has been a general trend since 2001 involving

---

10   Public Health Agency of Canada, 2017
11   Public Health Agency of Canada, 2017
12   Public Health Agency of Canada, 2017

an annual decrease of 2.1% in the age-standardized rate (ASR) of daily or occasional smokers in Canada.[13] While this is surely a step in the right direction, further action (whether it be a modified public health strategy or increased education on the topic) is needed to reduce the impact of smoking on the general health of the Canadian population, especially when we consider the potential effects of second-hand smoke that may be difficult to measure through public health data.

Next, physical inactivity is one of the most important public health concerns in the world, with the World Health Organization (WHO) identifying it as the fourth leading risk factor for chronic diseases and mortality worldwide.[14] In Canada, the recommendations for children and youth are to engage in at least 60 minutes of moderate to vigorous physical activity everyday while the recommendation for adults is to engage in 150 minutes of moderate-to-vigorous physical activity per week, with each bout lasting 10 minutes or more. However, 77.8% of Canadian adults and 90.7% of Canadian children did not meet the Canadian Physical Activity Guidelines in 2014, making physical inactivity a prominent health concern in Canada[15]. In general, the percentage of people who do not meet physical activity guidelines tends to increase from the younger age groups up to the older age groups, possibly due to increased time commitments needed for employment and other daily activities.

Related to physical inactivity is sedentary behaviour, which is defined as long periods of sitting that is usually done in conjunction with activities such as watching TV, playing video games, and using a computer.[16] Prolonged periods of sedentary activity can increase the risk of conditions such as obesity and negatively impact overall fitness. Studies have found that these associations are independent of physical activity, meaning that it is possible for someone who is physically active to still experience the same negative effects as

13   Public Health Agency of Canada, 2017
14   Public Health Agency of Canada, 2017
15   Public Health Agency of Canada, 2017
16   Public Health Agency of Canada, 2017

CHAPTER 1: THE MECHANISMS OF DIABETES

other people with similar sedentary activities who engage in less physical exercise. Some possible remedies for this issue include recommendations such as limiting recreational screen time to no more than 2 hours per day for children and youth.[17] However, it can be difficult to address sedentary behaviour caused by electronics due to the increasing popularity and importance of social media and other virtual/electronic forms of recreation in the 21st century.

Alcohol use in moderation is generally not severely harmful, but a significant proportion of Canadians aged 12 and older (17.9% or over 5.2 million) report heavy drinking on at least a monthly basis over the past year in 2014.[18] Binge or heavy drinking is generally defined as the consumption of 4 or more alcoholic drinks for women or 5 or more alcoholic drinks for men in a single occasion. There are immediate health impacts of binge or heavy drinking in addition to the risk of long-term excessive alcohol consumption, such as increased risk for diseases such as chronic liver disease and cancer, which may lead to premature death. Alcohol can also have impacts beyond chronic disease risk due to its sedative effects, such as its involvement in many motor vehicle accidents involving impaired driving.[19]

Finally, many Canadians have unhealthy diets in the sense that they do not consume adequate amounts of fruits and vegetables. Consuming the recommended number of servings of both fruits and vegetables can reduce the risk of diseases such as CVDs and cancer and generally lowers the risk of all-cause mortality.[20] While adequate fruit and vegetable consumption are not the sole components of a healthy diet, focusing on this aspect is useful for studying population-wide diets. According to Canada's Food Guide recommendations, adults should consume 7-10 servings of fruits and vegetables daily while children and youth should consume 4-8 servings. Unfortunately, around 60.3% of the Canadian population

---

17   Public Health Agency of Canada, 2017
18   Public Health Agency of Canada, 2017
19   Public Health Agency of Canada, 2017
20   Public Health Agency of Canada, 2017

aged 12 or older (around 17.1 million people) consumed fruits and vegetables less than five times a day according to 2014 data.[21] These findings could signify the need for further public education or outreach on health eating or policies that make fruits and vegetables more accessible and less expensive.

While relatively few Canadians have all four of the risk factors discussed above based on self-report data (only 2.3% of Canadians aged 20 years or older in 2014, for example), it is still concerning that the large majority of Canadians aged 20 years or older likely have at least one of the four risk factors.[22] For example, 2014 data showed that approximately 80.4% of Canadians 20 years or older had at least one risk factor. Even by themselves, each risk factor can have serious impacts on a person's health, especially from a long-term standpoint. While these four risk factors are not responsible for every instance of a chronic disease or health condition, public health interventions should continue to focus on these risk factors to improve the overall health of the Canadian population.

Additionally, there are two prominent risk conditions that greatly contribute to the development of other diseases: hypertension and obesity.[23] These two diseases are significant health issues in their own right due to their high prevalence and health impacts even before considering their impact on the development of other diseases. Hypertension, or high blood pressure, can cause cardiovascular effects such as reduced blood flow to certain organs and damaged arteries, which can lead to health conditions (such as stroke and heart attacks) and mortality. In 2012, approximately 24.9% of Canadians aged 20 years or older (around 6.9 million people) lived with diagnosed hypertension. Canada also has one of the highest, if not the highest national blood pressure control rates in the world at 68% of its population, further evidencing the severity of this issue. Obesity can increase the risk of conditions such as CVDs, certain forms of cancer, and premature death. Additionally,

21   Public Health Agency of Canada, 2017
22   Public Health Agency of Canada, 2017
23   Public Health Agency of Canada, 2017

it may also impact educational attainment, learning potential, and quality of life due to factors such as stigma.[24]

Health Inequalities

It is important to note inequalities or disparities that may exist in the rates and severity of health issues and risk factors across different groups within the general population and different geographic areas within Canada.

In the case of tobacco smoking, the Atlantic provinces (Newfoundland and Labrador, Prince Edward Island, Nova Scotia, New Brunswick) and territories (Yukon, the Northwest Territories and Nunavut) all had a proportion of daily or occasional smokers (measured using ASR) that was at least 20% above the national average.[25] In contrast, British Columbia had the lowest smoking rate at 14.4% in 2014. While there are obviously several factors or root causes behind this particular disparity, there is the potential for some of them (such as social customs and provincial regulations) to be addressed via education, policy changes, and other methods. Another example would be unhealthy eating, with the proportion of Canadians eating fruits and vegetables less than five times a day exceeding the national average by more than 20% in Newfoundland and Labrador (74.1% ASR) and Nunavut (76.6% ASR).[26]

It is important that we continue to gather the latest data and trends regarding these disparities in health conditions and risk factor prevalence through population-wide surveys or research. Following that, appropriate measures should be taken to address these disparities as they may allow us to improve the health of potentially vulnerable groups.

---

24   Public Health Agency of Canada, 2017
25   Public Health Agency of Canada, 2017
26   Public Health Agency of Canada, 2017

References

Health Canada, Background Document: Public Consultation on Strengthening Canada's Approach to Substance Use Issues (2018). Retrieved July 7, 2022, from https://www.canada.ca/en/health-canada/services/substance-use/canadian-drugs-substances-strategy/strengthening-canada-approach-substance-use-issue.html#a2.

Public Health Agency of Canada, How healthy are Canadians?: A trend analysis of the health of Canadians from a healthy living and chronic disease perspective (2017). Retrieved July 7, 2022, from https://www.canada.ca/en/public-health/services/publications/healthy-living/how-healthy-canadians.html#s2.

Lee, J., & Smith, J. P. (2018). Health, Economic Status, and Aging in High-Income Countries. In Future directions for the Demography of Aging: Proceedings of a workshop. essay, The National Academies Press.

Moroz, N., Moroz, I., & D'Angelo, M. S. (2020). Mental health services in Canada: Barriers and cost-effective solutions to increase access. *Healthcare management forum, 33*(6), 282–287. https://doi.org/10.1177/0840470420933911

Chapter 2: Cardiovascular Diseases in Canada

By Rebecca Tang

Introduction to Cardiovascular Diseases

Cardiology focuses on the study of the heart, a critical organ that solely functions to maintain adequate blood flow and nutrients to sustain the entire body. Diseases of the heart and blood vessels are classified under the general term called cardiovascular diseases (CVDs) or heart disease. CVDs are a global health concern and the second leading cause of death in Canada [1]. In Canada, CVDs are an imperative health issue as one-third of Canadians were reported to have died from CVDs and 16% of Canadians were hospitalized in 2009 [2]. Additionally, CVDs cost the Canadian' economy billions of dollars annually. It is a prevalent and relevant disease that can affect all Canadians by not discriminating against age, geography or ethnicity.

CVDs can be classified into four main types of heart diseases. The first is coronary artery disease or ischemic heart disease occurs when the arteries are narrowed or blocked causing heart attacks and angina. Ischemic heart disease is the most common type of CVD in Canada. Heart rhythm disorders is a second type of CVDs where the heart rhythm beats abnormally and can disrupt blood flow. One example of a heart rhythm disorder is tachycardia defined as rapid irregular heartbeats. Abnormalities of the heart valves, walls, or vessels are structural heart disease. Structural heart disease can be birth defects such as congenital heart disease and/or acquired through infections or other factors later in life. Lastly, heart failure is a serious condition that causes the physical heart to be weakened or become damaged and can no longer pump sufficient blood to the body.

CVDs impact the central organ in the body and can induce damage to other organ systems. While there are unmodifiable risk factors that can lead to CVD, there are many modifiable risk factors that can reduce the risk of CVD development. Unmodifiable risk factors including increased age, ethnicity, biological sex and family history are among the common risk factors [3,4]. Smoking, diet, exercise and lifestyle choices are modifiable risk factors that can contribute to reducing individuals' CVD risk [5]. The objective of this chapter is to provide an overview of CVD by highlighting the history of CVD, current epidemiology, treatment and future outlook in the Canadian content.

History of Cardiovascular Disease

CVD has been a complex and serious health concern for decades. In the 1920s, CVD was the leading cause of mortality in Canada [6]. It was estimated that half of dying Canadians died due to CVD in the 1950s [7]. Less than 20% of infants born with a heart defect reached adulthood in the 1950s [8]. The incidence of CVD has declined since the 1950s. Additionally, the total number of CVD deaths has been decreasing since 1979 despite the growing population in Canada [6]. The decrease can be attributed to various factors such as better preventive treatment, improved drug management or different lifestyle choices [9].

Various research milestones in cardiology have improved CVD patients' health outcomes over the years. For example, Dr. Wilfred Bigelow performed the first open-heart, which helped to increase patients with severe CVDs [9]. The technique became the standard practice of care throughout the 1950s. In the 1960s, the Toronto General Hospital established the first Canadian coronary care unit [10]. The coronary unit continues to be a renowned center for improving patients' health worldwide.

In the 1980s, advances in blood pressure research and identification of important biological molecular factors contributed to the improvement of cardiovascular health [11]. The Canadian Heart Health Initiative was launched in 1986 as a federal strategy to address health care costs and health concerns for Canadians [12]. In 1999, the Canadian Hypertension Education Program was launched to increase awareness of high blood pressure as a risk factor in CVDs [13]. Various advances in science and research enhanced the quality of life for patients with CVDs. However, it is predicted that a larger portion of susceptible individuals will become vulnerable to CVDs as the aging population grows older in the next decade.

Current epidemiology

CVDs are the second leading cause of all age disability-adjusted life years in Canada, only behind neoplasm between 2006 to 2016 [14]. In 2020, it was reported that CVDs took a total of about 53,704 deaths in Canada [15]. Men are more affected by CVD compared to women when compared at the time of death across all ages [15]. The sex differences diminish for people over the age of 85 years old [15].

A 2020 study found that the overall standardized hospitalization rates of CVD between 2007 and 2016 were 2.4% for heart failure, 4.7% for stroke and 27.4% for coronary artery disease [16]. These results suggest that the reduction in mortality risk has improved over time and can be attributed to improved treatment or management of CVDs. However, the same study found a 7.2% increase in the hospitalization rate for congenital heart disease [16]. Therefore, there are differences between CVD types and their impact on patients.

Nunavut has the lowest average CVD mortality of 97.2% per 100,000 population [17]. One possible explanation for the lower rate in Nunavut is the life expectancy in Nunavut is about 70 years old, which is relatively lower than the rest of Canada [17,18]. Therefore, residents in Nunavut may not live long enough to suffer from CVDs or other comorbidities leading to poor cardiovascular health. Newfoundland and Labrador ranked as the province with the highest CVDs rate with 320.6 occurrences per 100,000 in the population [19]. In comparison to 16 other international countries, Canada ranks 6th in cardiovascular mortality rank [17]. On average 141.1 Canadians died per 100,000 between 2009 and 2011 [17].

In the Public Health Agency of Canada 2010 report, diseases in the circulatory system cost the Canadian government about $13.6 billion [20]. The report emphasizes that circulatory system diseases' expenses are costly, especially for the older population with drug, patient care and hospital fees that continue to soar. The CVDs cost burden in Quebec is projected to increase by 100% if there are no lifestyle changes or technological advancements [21]. A study from Ontario reported missed preventive opportunities in primary care such as weight management and smoking habits that would improve cardiovascular health [22].

A study in Alberta reveals that patients at high risk for CVD can cost the healthcare system about $12,068 in the first-year of provincial treatment and decreases to about $4655 in the fifth year of the study [20]. It is estimated that for every $69 spent on cardiovascular care, $1 is invested into research efforts but for every $1 invested, it yields an annual benefit of $0.21 to the Canadian economy [23]. More investment into cardiovascular research would provide beneficial outcomes that would improve Canadians' health and relieve the economic burden.

Intervention and Treatment

The specific interventions and treatments for CVDs are dependent on the type of CVDs and the patient. Generally, more aggressive treatment options are reserved for patients with severe CVDs symptoms. Preventive measures against CVD are beneficial initial strategies to help avoid CVD development from the initial stages. Lifestyle choices such as physical activity, avoiding smoking, lower stress levels and reduction of alcohol have been shown to provide beneficial prevention and interventions against CVDs [24]. Additionally, lowering hypertension or high blood pressure is effective against stroke, coronary heart disease and heart failure [25]. Healthy diets consisting of at least 5 fruits or vegetables serving a day, low saturated fats and no processed carbohydrates will help prevent CVDs [26].

Patients with CVDs have various treatment options ranging from pharmacological, surgical and novel treatment options. In consultation with their healthcare professional, patients can have a single or combined treatment and management plans. Some common effective medication prescribed to patients with CVDs includes aspirin, β-blockers, statins or angiotensin-converting enzyme inhibitors [27]. Lowering cholesterol levels using statins is effective in preventing stroke and acute coronary syndrome [24]. Some operations that can be performed include coronary artery bypass, heart transplantation, valve repair or replacement. Targeted therapy is a promising area for precision medicine against CVDs. However, there are limitations such as off-target effects and genetic mutation that can be harmful to the patient in a clinical setting [28].

On the Horizon for Cardiovascular Diseases

While the overall mortality rates of CVDs have been decreasing, the burden of CVDs and future outlook may be worrisome. The high prevalence of obesity, diabetes and hypertension are growing concerns as these are risk factors that can lead to CVDs [16]. It highlights the increased demand to investigate more effective actions for the prevention and management of these risk factors.

Physical activity is one effective preventive factor against CVDs with an inverse dose-dependent relationship [29,30]. Canadians who exercise for at least 150 minutes of moderate physical activity a week have a 14% reduction in CVD risk compared to Canadians who are inactive [16,31]. The COVID-19 pandemic has enforced restrictions on Canadians and impacted physical activity opportunities with gym and park closure. Stay-at-home restrictions can have long-term effects and increase CVDs risk for Canadians in the future.

People who meet the recommended physical activity guidelines have a 10.6% increased risk of CVDs development when their physical activity reduces by 40% [32]. Similar to people who do not meet the physical activity recommendation, there is a 4.3% increase when physical activity decreases by 40% [32]. However, for people who exceeded the recommendation before COVID-19, their cardiovascular risk does not change with decreased physical activity [32]. Therefore, it is expected that decreased physical activity during the COVID-19 pandemic can have long-term effects and contribute to the increased CVDs incidence.

References

1.   Canada PHA of. Heart Disease in Canada [Internet]. 2017 [cited 2022 Jul 8]. Available from: https://www.canada.ca/en/public-health/services/publications/diseases-conditions/heart-disease-canada.html

2.   Smith ER. The Canadian Heart Health Strategy and Action Plan. Can J Cardiol. 2009 Aug;25(8):451–2.

3.   Cardiovascular disease risk factors [Internet]. Ada. [cited 2022 Jul 8]. Available from: https://ada.com/cardiovascular-disease-risk-factors/

4.   Mancini GBJ, Gosselin G, Chow B, Kostuk W, Stone J, Yvorchuk KJ, et al. Canadian Cardiovascular Society Guidelines for the Diagnosis and Management of Stable Ischemic Heart Disease. Canadian Journal of Cardiology. 2014 Aug;30(8):837–49.

5.   Beyond Established and Novel Risk Factors | Circulation [Internet]. [cited 2022 Jul 8]. Available from: https://www.ahajournals.org/doi/10.1161/circulationaha.107.738732

6.   Nair C, Colburn H, McLean D, Petrasovits A. Cardiovascular disease in Canada. Health Rep. 1989;1(1):1–22.

7.   Nicholls ES, Jung J. Cardiovascular disease mortality in Canada. 1950;12.

8.   Reid GJ, Webb GD, Barzel M, McCrindle BW, Irvine MJ, Siu SC. Estimates of Life Expectancy by Adolescents and Young Adults With Congenital Heart Disease. Journal of the American College of Cardiology. 2006 Jul 18;48(2):349–55.

9.   Kermode-Scott B. Wilfred G Bigelow. BMJ. 2005 Apr 23;330(7497):967.

10.   Lee MM, Alvarez J, Rao V. History of Cardiovascular Surgery at Toronto General Hospital. Seminars in Thoracic and Cardiovascular Surgery. 2016 Sep 1;28(3):700–4.

11.   Kotchen TA. Historical Trends and Milestones in Hypertension Research. Hypertension. 2011 Oct;58(4):522–38.

12.   Preventing Chronic Disease: April 2007: 06_0076 [Internet]. [cited 2022 Jul 8]. Available from: https://www.cdc.gov/pcd/issues/2007/apr/06_0076.htm

13.   McAlister FA, Wooltorton E, Campbell NRC. The Canadian Hypertension Education Program (CHEP) recommendations: launching a new series. CMAJ. 2005 Aug 30;173(5):508–9.

14.   Global Burden of Disease Study trends for Canada from 1990 to 2016 | CMAJ [Internet]. [cited 2022 Jul 8]. Available from: https://www.cmaj.ca/content/190/44/E1296

15.   Government of Canada SC. Leading causes of death, total population, by age group [Internet]. 2022 [cited 2022 Jul 8]. Available from: https://www150.statcan.gc.ca/t1/tbl1/en/tv.action?pid=1310039401

16.   Botly LCP, Lindsay MP, Mulvagh SL, Hill MD, Goia C, Martin-Rhee M, et al. Recent Trends in Hospitalizations for Cardiovascular Disease, Stroke, and Vascular Cognitive Impairment in Canada. Canadian Journal of Cardiology. 2020 Jul 1;36(7):1081–90.

17.   Mortality Due to Heart Disease and Stroke [Internet]. Conference Board. [cited 2022 Jul 6]. Available from: https://www.conferenceboard.ca/hcp/provincial/health/heart.aspx

18.   Government of Canada SC. The Daily — Deaths, 2019 [Internet]. 2020 [cited 2022 Jul 8]. Available from: https://www150.statcan.gc.ca/n1/daily-quotidien/201126/dq201126b-eng.htm

19.   Kreatsoulas C, Anand SS. The impact of social determinants on cardiovascular disease. Can J Cardiol. 2010;26(Suppl C):8C-13C.

20.   Canada PHA of. Economic Burden of Illness in Canada, 2010 [Internet]. 2018 [cited 2022 Jul 8]. Available from: https://www.canada.ca/en/public-health/services/publications/science-research-data/economic-burden-illness-canada-2010.html

21.   Boisclair D, Décarie Y, Laliberté-Auger F, Michaud PC, Vincent C. The economic benefits of reducing cardiovascular disease mortality in Quebec, Canada. PLOS ONE. 2018 Jan 4;13(1):e0190538.

22.   Liddy C, Singh J, Hogg W, Dahrouge S, Deri-Armstrong C, Russell G, et al. Quality of cardiovascular disease care in Ontario, Canada: missed opportunities for prevention - a cross sectional study. BMC Cardiovascular Disorders. 2012 Sep 12;12(1):74.

23.   Oliveira C de, Nguyen HV, Wijeysundera HC, Wong WWL, Woo G, Grootendorst P, et al. Estimating the payoffs from cardiovascular disease research in Canada: an economic analysis. Canadian Medical Association Open Access Journal. 2013 May 16;1(2):E83–90.

24.   Leong DP, Joseph PG, McKee M, Anand SS, Teo KK, Schwalm JD, et al. Reducing the Global Burden of Cardiovascular Disease, Part 2. Circulation Research. 2017 Sep;121(6):695–710.

25.   Ettehad D, Emdin CA, Kiran A, Anderson SG, Callender T, Emberson J, et al. Blood pressure lowering for prevention of cardiovascular disease and death: a systematic review and meta-analysis. Lancet. 2016 Mar 5;387(10022):957–67.

26.   Tobe SW, Stone JA, Brouwers M, Bhattacharyya O, Walker KM, Dawes M, et al. Harmonization of guidelines for the prevention and treatment of cardiovascular disease: the C-CHANGE Initiative. CMAJ. 2011 Oct 18;183(15):E1135–50.

27.   Cardiovascular diseases (CVDs) [Internet]. [cited 2022 Jul 8]. Available from: https://www.who.int/news-room/fact-sheets/detail/cardiovascular-diseases-(cvds)

28.   Xu M, Song J. Targeted Therapy in Cardiovascular Disease: A Precision Therapy Era. Front Pharmacol. 2021 Apr 16;12:623674.

29.   Ross R, Chaput JP, Giangregorio LM, Janssen I, Saunders TJ, Kho ME, et al. Canadian 24-Hour Movement Guidelines for Adults aged 18-64 years and Adults aged 65 years or older: an integration of physical activity, sedentary behaviour, and sleep. Appl Physiol Nutr Metab. 2020 Oct;45(10 (Suppl. 2)):S57–102.

30.   Sattelmair J, Pertman J, Ding EL, Kohl HW, Haskell W, Lee IM. Dose response between physical activity and risk of coronary heart disease: a meta-analysis. Circulation. 2011 Aug 16;124(7):789–95.

31.   Arem H, Moore SC, Patel A, Hartge P, Berrington de Gonzalez A, Visvanathan K, et al. Leisure Time Physical Activity and Mortality: A Detailed Pooled Analysis of the Dose-Response Relationship. JAMA Internal Medicine. 2015 Jun 1;175(6):959–67.

32.   Government of Canada SC. The effect of COVID-19 on physical activity among Canadians and the future risk of cardiovascular disease [Internet]. 2021 [cited 2022 Jul 8]. Available from: https://www150.statcan.gc.ca/n1/pub/45-28-0001/2021001/article/00019-eng.htm

Chapter 3: What is Diabetes mellitus, and where did it originate?

By Aida Zaheer

Diabetes mellitus is a disease which has been known since Antiquity. It is a group of chronic, metabolic diseases characterized by hyperglycemia, which encompasses elevated blood glucose levels (Karamanou et al., 2016). The main types of diabetes to be discussed throughout this chapter are Type 1 and Type 2 diabetes, which are known as insulin-dependent and adult-onset diabetes, respectively (WHO, 2022).

The origin of Diabetes can be traced back to around 250 BC, when Araetus of Cappadocia first coined the term "diabetes". The addition of the term "mellitus", which means "sweet" in Latin, was later added in 1675 by Thoman Willis, who aimed to further accurately describe this disease by the extremely sweet taste of its urine (Awad, 2022). However, it's important to note that this particularly discovery was not originally found by Willis, but was instead discovered by the famous Indian surgeon Sushruta, approximately during the 5th century BC (Karamanou et al., 2016)

Despite the recognition received by all the aforementioned historical figures who helped pave the way to the discovery of diabetes, it is the Ancient Egyptians, Chinese, Indians and Arabs who have failed to receive recognition for their initial attempts to clinically establish the symptoms and signs of diabetes (Karamanou et al., 2016).

How does Diabetes affect the whole body?

As a chronic disease, the sustained levels of hyperglycemia that encompass diabetes can lead to serious heart, nerve and kidney damage over time (WHO, 2022). These long term complications develop gradually, and can eventually be disabling and even life-threatening to diabetic individuals- let's begin by delving into the specific outcomes of these complications.

Diabetes and heart diseases often go hand-in-hand. It is known to drastically increase risks of cardiovascular complications, including coronary artery disease, chest pains (clinically defined as angina), strokes, and heart attacks (Mayo Clinic, 2020). These risks are primarily exacerbated by the damage that Diabetes has on the blood vessels that control our hearts (cite same link as above).

In addition to damaging blood vessels, the excess blood sugar caused by Diabetes can injure the walls of capillaries that nourish our nerves within various parts of the body, including our legs and heart (Mayo Clinic, 2020). This is termed as Neuropathy, which tends to cause a burning sensation, numbness and tingling feeling that spreads throughout the body, eventually leading to a loss of all sense of feeling in the affected limbs, if left untreated.

Finally, the effects of Diabetes can damage glomeruli- the tiny blood vessel clusters as part of the kidneys, that filter waste from blood. Damage to this filtration system can be severe enough to cause kidney failure and subsequently the need for a kidney transplant or dialysis (Mayo Clinic, 2020).

Type 1 Diabetes Mellitus

Type 1 Diabetes Mellitus (T1DM), also known as Insulin-dependent diabetes, is a genetic disorder that occurs due to lack of insulin production by the pancreas (CDC, 2022). More specifically, the lack of insulin occurs due to the destruction of the insulin-producing pancreatic beta cells. As a result, people with Type 1 Diabetes require life-long therapy for insulin replacement (Lucier & Weinstock, 2022).

Insulin is an anabolic hormone that is vital to carry out the processes of storing glucose as glycogen in the liver (glycogenesis), the synthesis of fatty acids, inhibiting fat breakdown in adipose tissue (lipolysis), and importantly stimulating glucose entry into muscles and adipose cells.

Without this vital hormone, individuals with T1DM are prone to developing diabetic ketoacidosis - a serious complication of diabetes that can become life-threatening (Lucier & Weinstock, 2022).

Since individuals with T1DM cannot produce insulin themselves due to destruction of pancreatic beta cells, they must take insulin themselves as a form of treatment therapy (Mayo Clinic, 2022). Beyond this, supplemental treatment forms include monitoring blood glucose levels often, having a healthy diet, exercising frequently and counting the dietary intake of carbohydrates, proteins and fats (Mayo Clinic, 2022).

Type 2 Diabetes Mellitus

Type 2 Diabetes Mellitus (T2DM), formerly known as adult-onset diabetes, is a long-term condition that impairs the ways in which the body uses blood glucose as a source of fuel (Mayo Clinic, 2021). It results in blood sugar levels that are too elevated and that can, eventually result in the development of disorders within the nervous, circulatory and immune systems (Mayo Clinic, 2021). Similarly to T1DM, this disease results due to an impairment in the availability of insulin from pancreatic beta cells. However, the causes stem from 2 interrelated problems- the pancreas doesn't produce enough insulin to sustain the regulation of glucose entry into the cell, and cells respond poorly to the available insulin, thus they take in less sugar (Mayo Clinic, 2021).

As mentioned, this type of Diabetes Mellitus was formerly known as "adult-onset" diabetes, but is no longer referred to by that title, due to its ability to be present during both childhood and adulthood years of life (Mayo Clinic, 2021). Despite being more commonly found within the adult population, its prevalence is increasing within the younger generation. Specifically, there has been an increase in T2DM within the subset of children who are obese (Mayo Clinic, 2021).

Despite treatment recommendations that encompass lifestyle changes, such as exercising more frequently, taking diabetes medication or insulin therapy to regulate blood glucose levels, eating healthier and losing weight, there is no established "cure" for the complete remission of T2DM (Mayo Clinic, 2021).

Gestational Diabetes

Gestational Diabetes is a type of diabetes that is diagnosed for the first time during a pregnancy (gestation). Similarly to T1DM and T2DM, it affects the ways in which body cells utilize glucose (Mayo Clinic, 2022). Since this type of Diabetes occurs during a pregnancy, sustained high levels of blood glucose pose effects on the pregnancy that can put the baby's health at risk (Mayo Clinic, 2022).

During pregnancy, insulin resistance can occur as a result of bodily changes that make the body use insulin less effectively. Changes such as weight gain contribute to the buildup of insulin resistance, ultimately increasing the body's need for insulin (CDC, 2021). This insulin resistance is bound to occur within the pregnancies of all pregnant women to some degree, however some women have insulin resistance before their pregnancy, thus increasing their risk of developing gestational diabetes, due to their elevated need for insulin (CDC, 2021). Nearly 50% of pregnant women with gestational diabetes later develop T2DM, however prevention methods can be put in place to minimize the risk of this development happening (CDC, 2021).

Luckily, this type of Diabetes Mellitus can be easily managed by getting regular physical activity, monitoring the baby, checking blood sugar levels and eating healthy foods, to ensure preservation of the mother and baby's health (CDC, 2021).

The Demographic Prevalence: Impacts on North American Countries

Currently, 37.3 million (11.3%) people across the US population have diabetes; 28.7 million of those individuals being diagnosed and 8.5 million of those individuals remaining undiagnosed (CDC, 2022). Additionally, 96 million (38%) of the adult population (aged 18 years or older) in the US have prediabetes, along with 26.4 million (48.8%) people aged 64 or older within the US have prediabetes (CDC, 2022). These shocking numbers display the increased prevalence and risk of diabetes that has become heavily normalized at the national level, within the US.

Similarly, diabetes rates within Canada continue to climb, showing no signs of decreasing or leveling. Currently, more than 5.7 million (10%) Canadians are living with diagnosed T1DM or T2DM (Diabetes Canada, 2022). Additionally, there are 11.7 million (30%) Canadians living with either Diabetes or Prediabetes; these individuals are at risk of developing T2DM if left unmanaged (Diabetes Canada, 2022).

Within the IDF North America and Caribbean Region, there are currently 51 million adults, aged 20 to 79 years old, living with diabetes (IDF, 2021). These high figures are expected to continue increasing up to 57 million by 2030 and even 63 million by 2045 (IDF, 2021). Additionally, there are 12 million adults aged 20 to 79 years old, living with undiagnosed diabetes. Regarding individuals with pre-diabetic conditions within this region, 47 million adults aged 20 to 79 years old have impaired glucose tolerance, putting them at a high risk of developing T2DM, if these conditions are left unmanaged (IDF, 2021). Finally, statistics exhibit that 1 in 6 live births within the IDF North America and Caribbean Region are affected by hyperglycemia throughout the pregnancy, contributing to the negative consequences of gestational diabetes experienced by pregnant women (IDF, 2021).

Overall, Diabetes is affecting 422 million people worldwide, with this number particularly affecting populations of individuals living in low and middle income countries. Each year, around 1.5 million deaths are attributed directly to Diabetes, with both of these figures steadily increasing throughout the past decades (WHO, 2022).

The Costly Impact of Diabetes

Beyond the health impacts that accompany Diabetes, financial burden can result from a lack of management of this disease. According to the American Diabetes Association (ADA), the cost of diabetes has risen 26% over a five year period, rising from $245 billion in 2012 to $327 billion in 2017 (ADA, 2018). A breakdown of these figures show that the largest portion of these costs can be attributed to medical costs. Specifically, these expenditures encompass 30% hospital inpatient care costs, 30% prescription costs to treat diabetes complications, 15% the cost of anti-diabetic supplies and 13% physician office visits (ADA, 2018). On average, individuals who have diabetes incur medical expenditures that are on average 2.3 times higher than medical expenditures in the absence of diabetes (ADA, 2018).

These estimates show the substantial impacts faced by society as a result of Diabetes, due to the heavy financial burden being placed on individuals living with the risk of health complications that accompany Diabetes. According to the American costs of diabetes in specific populations, most costs of Diabetes care within the US (i.e. 67.3%), can be covered by government insurance, while the rest of the cost is either paid by uninsured individuals (2%), or private insurance (30.7%) (ADA, 2018). Evidently, this poses higher health risks to the lower income, uninsured individuals living with Diabetes, due to the financial disparities faced by this subset population.

The Disparities faced by High-Risk Populations

The incidence and cost rates of diabetes are in many ways tied to racial and socio-economic disparities faced by high-risk populations across North America. These populations face a disproportionately higher risk of diabetes, rates of complications tied to diabetes, and mortality due to diabetes (Hill-Briggs et al., 2020).

Diabetes disproportionately affects African Americans, Latinos/ Hispanics and Asian Americans, posing 77%, 66% and 18% higher risk of having a diabetes diagnosis compared to their white adult counterparts, respectively (Meng et al., 2016). These racial minority groups are less likely to receive recommended diabetes services and additionally, receive lower quality of care along with greater self-management barriers (Meng et al., 2016). As a result, these groups face more disproportionate health impacts that make the management of this disease significantly more difficult to maintain and afford (Meng et al., 2016).

The Social Determinants of Health furthermore show that socio-economic status (SES) heavily influences diabetes-related health outcomes (Hill-Briggs et al., 2020). Individuals who are lower on the SES ladder are proven to be more likely to develop T2DM, be at a greater risk of death as a result of Diabetes, and are bound to experience more diabetes-related complications compared to those higher up on the SES ladder (Hill-Briggs et al., 2020). If an individual attains a higher SES, they receive a higher income, are likely to have a greater level of educational attainment, have a higher occupational grade and subsequently, be at a lower risk of developing T2DM or experiencing its related complications (Hill-Briggs et al., 2020).

The Need for Treatment

In order to subsidize the financial and health-related costs associated with diabetes, Governments must begin by taking a lead on the implementation of decision support tools, to aid in diabetes management (Diabetes Canada, 2022). Furthermore, it is important for Governments across North America to adopt Nationwide approaches, in order to reduce the out-of-pocket costs for people living with diabetes, that pertain specifically to groups facing racial/ethnic and SES disparities. By doing so, more healthcare resources can be presented to high-risk populations, making it easier for them to manage the healthcare effects of Diabetes and subsequently, aids in the long term reduction of Diabetes across North American countries.

References

ADA. (2018, March). The cost of diabetes. The Cost of Diabetes | American Diabetes Association. Retrieved July 10, 2022, from https://www.diabetes.org/about-us/statistics/cost-diabetes

Awad, A. M. (2022, April 23). History of diabetes mellitus. Saudi medical journal. Retrieved July 10, 2022, from https://pubmed.ncbi.nlm.nih.gov/11953758/#:~:text=The%20term%20%22diabetes%22%20was%20first,noticed%20by%20the%20ancient%20Indians)

CDC. (2021, August 10). Gestational diabetes. Centers for Disease Control and Prevention. Retrieved July 10, 2022, from https://www.cdc.gov/diabetes/basics/gestational.html

CDC. (2022, January 18). National Diabetes Statistics Report. Centers for Disease Control and Prevention. Retrieved July 10, 2022, from https://www.cdc.gov/diabetes/data/statistics-report/index.html

CDC. (2022, March 11). What is type 1 diabetes? Centers for Disease Control and Prevention. Retrieved July 10, 2022, from https://www.cdc.gov/diabetes/basics/what-is-type-1-diabetes.html

Diabetes Canada. (2022, February). Diabetes in Canada: Backgrounder. Ottawa: Diabetes Canada. Retrieved July 10, 2022, from https://www.diabetes.ca/DiabetesCanadaWebsite/media/Advocacy-and-Policy/Backgrounder/2022_Backgrounder_Canada_English_1.pdf

Diabetes Canada. (2022, March). Diabetes rates continue to climb in Canada. DiabetesCanadaWebsite. Retrieved July 10, 2022, from https://www.diabetes.ca/media-room/press-releases/diabetes-rates-continue-to-climb-in-canada

Hill-Briggs, F., Adler, N. E., Berkowitz, S. A., Chin, M. H., Gary-Webb, T. L., Navas-Acien, A., Thornton, P. L., & Haire-Joshu, D. (2020, November 2). Social Determinants of Health and diabetes: A scientific review. American Diabetes Association. Retrieved July 10, 2022, from https://diabetesjournals.org/care/article/44/1/258/33180/Social-Determinants-of-Health-and-Diabetes-A

IDF. (2021, December). Diabetes in NAC. International Diabetes Federation. Retrieved July 10, 2022, from https://www.idf.org/our-network/regions-members/north-america-and-caribbean/diabetes-in-nac.html

Karamanou, M., Protogerou, A., Tsoucalas, G., Androutsos, G., & Poulakou-Rebelakou, E. (2016, January 10). Milestones in the history of diabetes mellitus: The main contributors. World journal of diabetes. Retrieved July 10, 2022, from https://www.ncbi.nlm.nih.gov/pmc/articles/PMC4707300/

Lucier , J., & Weinstock, R. S. (2022, January). Diabetes mellitus type 1. National Center for Biotechnology Information. Retrieved July 10, 2022, from https://pubmed.ncbi.nlm.nih.gov/29939535/

Mayo Clinic. (2020, October 30). Diabetes. Mayo Clinic. Retrieved July 10, 2022, from https://www.mayoclinic.org/diseases-conditions/diabetes/symptoms-causes/syc-20371444#:~:text=Diabetes%20dramatically%20increases%20the%20risk,Nerve%20damage%20(neuropathy)

Mayo Clinic. (2021, January 20). Type 2 diabetes. Mayo Clinic. Retrieved July 10, 2022, from https://www.mayoclinic.org/diseases-conditions/type-2-diabetes/symptoms-causes/syc-20351193#:~:text=Overview,circulatory%2C%20nervous%20and%20immune%20systems

Mayo Clinic. (2022, April 9). Gestational diabetes. Mayo Clinic. Retrieved July 10, 2022, from https://www.mayoclinic.org/diseases-conditions/gestational-diabetes/symptoms-causes/syc-20355339#:~:text=Gestational%20diabetes%20is%20diabetes%20diagnosed,pregnancy%20and%20your%20baby's%20health

Mayo Clinic. (2022, July 7). Type 1 diabetes. Mayo Clinic. Retrieved July 10, 2022, from https://www.mayoclinic.org/diseases-conditions/type-1-diabetes/diagnosis-treatment/drc-20353017

Meng, Y.-Y., Diamant, A., Jones, J., Lin, W., Chen, X., Wu, S.-H., Pourat, N., Roby, D., & Kominski, G. F. (2016, March 10). Racial and ethnic disparities in diabetes care and impact of vendor-based disease management programs. American Diabetes Association. Retrieved July 10, 2022, from https://diabetesjournals.org/care/article/39/5/743/30624/Racial-and-Ethnic-Disparities-in-Diabetes-Care-and

WHO. (2022). Diabetes. World Health Organization. Retrieved July 10, 2022, from https://www.who.int/health-topics/diabetes#tab=tab_1

Chapter 4: Obesity

By Lilian Yeung

An introduction to obesity and what it is

Obesity has long been considered a great concern for health officials as it continues to rise in Canada. It is a cumulative chronic disease in which excessive fat is accumulated on the body to the point of detrimental health. A common method of determining obesity is by using Body Mass Index (BMI) whereby a person's weight and height are taken into account to obtain their BMI. As such, this would give a basic overview of whether this person falls into the category of obese. But health officials and clinicians use much more than just BMI when clinically diagnosinng someone as obese.

There are many factors related to obesity and whether a person has a higher likelihood of obtaining it. Variables such as genetics, fat metabolism, physical activity levels, eating habits, sociodemographic, perception of healthy foods, social support, trauma, and many more all play a role in determining a person's disposition for obesity.

Trajectory of Obesity

Before a person reaches obesity, they are first overweight and this is something that has been noted as an increasing trend in the past century. According to a 1953 Canadian weight-height survey, which was conducted to convey the current situation and provide a reference for future studies, it highlighted the need for concern over the rising trends of excessive adipose tissues (Pett et al., 1956). This survey was the first representative survey of both body mass and height conducted on a national level (Katzmarzyk, P. T., 2012). As of now, there are no structured record-tracking of Canada's population and the prevalence of obesity based on body mass and height (Katzmarzyk, P. T., 2012).

Currently, rates of adult obesity prevalence in Canada has been projected to continue its incline within the following two decades (Bancej et al., 2015). This is a concerning trend as research has indicated that about a quarter of Canadian adults are obese and about 1 in 7 teenagers and children arre obese Bancej et al., 2015). Though obesity rates for Canadian children and adolescents have remained relatively stable since 2007 with no significant increases, this may change due to the quarantine period Bancej et al., 2015). Furthermore, the projected increase of obesity rates will be more prevalent in males than females throughout all stages of life (Bancej et al., 2015).

Possible factors relating to obesity and the rise of it

A possible explanation for the rising prevalence of excessive adipose may be attributed to the industrialization and processing of foods along with the increased access to foods. It has been noted for quite some time that ultra processed food—defined as foods containing industrial formulations such as cosmetic additives (artificial coloring/flavoring) and limited quantities of whole foods—do not have as much nutrition as whole foods (Rauber's 1st source). Common examples of ultra processed foods can be found in almost all countries ranging from first to third world countries following the ever-expanding reach of fast foods and chain restaurants that heavily sell processed food. Examples of processed foods include soft drinks or pop, candy, chips, pre-made frozen meals, packaged breads/buns, and products including reconstituted meat. Through the procedure of processing foods, it allows a longer shelf life, giving it more flavor that appeals to people. Furthermore, the convenience, large package sizes, aggressive media and advertisements, along with its affordable price of these processed foods ensures that most people, especially those with a lower socioeconomic background, would be consuming a lot more processed foods than whole foods. Numerous studies have demonstrated that consumption of processed foods has been linked with increased weight leading to a higher risk of being overweight and obesity. Processed foods is a world-wide problem that many countries are facing besides Canada. In the UK alone, several studies have shown a strong link between the consumption of ultra-processed foods and the dietary intake profiles of individuals with obesity (Raubner et al., 2021). A 2019 study analyzing the Canadian population by Nardocci et al. highlighted the correlation between consumption of ultra-processed food and obesity. By analyzing adults aged 18 years or more, they noted their BMI and estimated their ultra-processed food consumption through food recalls for the past 24 hours. Possible confounding variables were taken into account such as physical activity, socio-demographic, geographical location, smoking, and self-reported vs. measured weight and height. Nardocci et al. concluded that Canadians should reduce their intake of ultra-processed products accompanying additional consumption of fresh foods and dishes using unprocessed or limited amounts of processed foods.

Compounding the effects of ultra-processed foods is the fact that there is an upward trend in sedentary behavior due a mix of sedentary jobs as well as sedentary hobbies (such as media consumption via Instagram, Facebook, TikTok, Snapchat, etc.). With the rise of technological advancements and usage, there is a noticeable lack of physical activity or exercise by people due to the ease and convenience of their devices along with the instant gratification that comes along with using electronic devices (Rosen et al., 2014). Consistent research has shown that adolescents, teenagers, and children that use excessive amounts of screen time and media develop a higher disposition towards obesity, less physical activity, and overall poor health (Rosen et al., 2014). The study by Rosen et al. in 2014 illustrated that almost all technology activity has predicted decreased health for teenagers. As such, research indicates that setting limits and boundaries are necessary for the usage of technology for teenagers, adolescents, and children. Adults can also benefit from setting boundaries and limits for their screen usage as they are also susceptible to the risks associated with extensive screen time and media consumption. Moreover, healthy eating habits and physical activity are necessary in order to maintain good health.

Although healthy habits including eating whole foods with minimal processing in dishes is encouraged, not all demographics are able to access such foods. Barriers to eating healthy typically apply to those of a lower socioeconomic background and those with limited access to fresh foods based on their geography. Because of the streamlined processing of foods along with the higher prices of fresh foods, it limits people from a lower socioeconomic background to choose processing foods over fresh foods as they are forced to choose quantity over quality for their food. Furthermore, family, friends, and peers play a significant role in the choices we make regarding our food. In the case of children and dependents living with parents or legal guardians, they often do not get the option of choosing what to eat or how their food is prepared. Peer pressure and society also dictates what we consume. For example, people have a tendency of wanting to portray a certain image or fitting in or appeasing others, so they may partake in overconsumption of alcohol in social settings. Geographical location is also an impactful barrier to accessing fresh foods, especially for those who are unable to afford the time and resources to access fresh foods. Oftentimes, Indigenous peoples living in residential areas or remote locations have an especially hard time accessing fresh food and the full benefit of fresh foods due to the increased cost of fresh foods compared to processed foods. The increased cost is likely due to the transporting of food to remote/residential areas and as a result, the quality of fresh foods is also negatively affected. As such, Indigenous peoples are faced with the issue between choosing processed foods that are cheaper, greater portion size, and lasts longer than fresh foods.

Triggers for Obesity

There are also many possible situational or environmental triggers for obesity. Such triggers may include a sudden traumatic event occurring or stress.

References

https://obesitycanada.ca/obesity-in-canada/

https://www.proquest.com/docview/1301822415/
fulltextPDF/64F662A48DA149B1PQ/1?accountid=15115
- Pett, L. B., Ogilvie, G. F. (1956) The Canadian Weight-Height Survey. *Hum Biol 28:* 177– 188.
- In-text citation: (Pett et al., 1956)

https://onlinelibrary.wiley.com/doi/full/10.1038/oby.2002.90
Katzmarzyk, P.T. (2002), The Canadian Obesity Epidemic: An Historical Perspective. *Obesity Research, 10:* 666-674. https://doi.org/10.1038/oby.2002.90
- In-text citation: (Katzmarzyk, P. T., 2012)

https://onlinelibrary.wiley.com/action/
showCitFormats?doi=10.1038%2Foby.2001.123
- James, P.T., Leach, R., Kalamara, E. and Shayeghi, M. (2001), The Worldwide Obesity Epidemic. *Obesity Research, 9:* 228S-233S. https://doi.org/10.1038/oby.2001.123
- In-text citation: (James et al., 2001)

https://www.ncbi.nlm.nih.gov/pmc/articles/PMC100878/
- Katzmarzyk P. T. (2002). The Canadian obesity epidemic, 1985-1998. CMAJ : Canadian Medical Association journal = journal de l'Association medicale canadienne, 166(8), 1039–1040.
- In-text citation: (Katzmarzyk, P. T., 2002)

https://www.ncbi.nlm.nih.gov/pmc/articles/PMC4910458/
- Bancej, C., Jayabalasingham, B., Wall, R. W., Rao, D. P., Do, M. T., de Groh, M., & Jayaraman, G. C. (2015). Evidence Brief--Trends and projections of obesity among Canadians. *Health promotion and chronic disease prevention in Canada : research, policy and practice, 35*(7), 109–112. https://doi.org/10.24095/hpcdp.35.7.02

- In-text citation: (Bancej et al., 2015)

https://link.springer.com/article/10.1007/s00394-020-02367-1#citeas
- Rauber, F., Chang, K., Vamos, E.P. et al. Ultra-processed food consumption and risk of obesity: a prospective cohort study of UK Biobank. Eur J Nutr 60, 2169–2180 (2021). https://doi.org/10.1007/s00394-020-02367-1
- In-text citation: (Rauber et al., 2021)

https://link.springer.com/article/10.17269/s41997-018-0130-x
- Nardocci, M., Leclerc, BS., Louzada, ML. et al. Consumption of ultra-processed foods and obesity in Canada. Can J Public Health 110, 4–14 (2019). https://doi.org/10.17269/s41997-018-0130-x
- In-text citation: (Nardocci et al., 2019)

https://www.ncbi.nlm.nih.gov/pmc/articles/PMC4338000/#:~:text=Further%2C%20research%20shows%20that%20children,physical%20activity%2C%20and%20decreased%20health.
- Rosen, L. D., Lim, A. F., Felt, J., Carrier, L. M., Cheever, N. A., Lara-Ruiz, J. M., Mendoza, J. S., & Rokkum, J. (2014). Media and technology use predicts ill-being among children, preteens and teenagers independent of the negative health impacts of exercise and eating habits. Computers in human behavior, 35, 364–375. https://doi.org/10.1016/j.chb.2014.01.036
- In-text citation: (Rosen et al., 2014)

Chapter 5: Parkinson's Disease

By Francis Fernandes

History

Parkinson's Disease (PD) is most prevalent neurodegenerative disease whose chronicity and progressiveness are characterized by motor/non-motor features.[1] PD was first clinically described by a British physician named Dr. James Parkinson in an essay published in the 1817.[2] In its early stages of discovery and discussion, PD was referred to "shaking palsy" and defined as;

> *"Involuntary tremulous motion, with lessened voluntary power, in parts not in action, and even when supported; with a propensity to bend the trunk forwards, and to pass from a walking to a running pace: the senses and intellects being uninjured."* [3]

Parkinson's early essay on PD included six case studies in patients, three of whom were captured from observations individuals seen at a distance on the streets of London during the early 1800s.[2] A more thorough description was published 50 years after James Parkinson's initial work by Jean-Martin Charcot, a prominent French neurologist .[2] In a series of then published lectures, Charcot began to differentiate clinical subtypes and associate symptoms that accompany the disease. Charcot was also the first to use/establish the term PD as a mode of rejecting James Parkinson's early description of "shaking palsy".[4] Since Charcot's initial findings, French neurologists were at the forefront of clinically observing, describing, and reporting relevant information regarding PD.

The pathophysiological basis for the development of PD and associated symptoms were largely investigated during early and mid 1900s. Joseph Babinski, a French-Polish neurologist was one of the first to attribute the distinct motor fluctuations of PD (i.e., tremors) to the substantia nigra, [5] an neuroanatomical region vital for physical movement control and dopamine production.[1] It was not until second part of the 20th century that the world received a robust catalogue of PD, including a staging system for the development of PD. Heohn and Year's publication in 1967 paved the way for a globally recognized and utilized scale which quantified an understanding of PD and its prognosis. It also revolutionized the diagnostic process of PD and introduced the importance of early detection and treatment for the management of PD.[2]

Treatments for PD were often investigated in tandem with the diagnostic efforts of PD. James Parkinson's essay on "shaking palsy" advocated for the then widespread modality of blood-letting, which he postulated reduced inflammatory pressure in the brain and spinal cord, thus reducing the tremor-like symptoms.[2] In addition to Charcot's investigations on the presentation of PD, he was also deeply involved with studying the efficacy of existing pharmacological agents for management of PD. The overwhelmingly poor efficacy of these agents were described in the below statement:

> *"Everything, or almost everything, has been tried against this disease. Among the medicinal substances that have been extolled and which I have myself administered to no avail, I need only enumerate a few…"* [4]

In response to the poor outcomes of poor pharmacological interventions at the time, Charcot opted for a modality-based approach of involving vibration. In the latter part of the 1800s, Charcot commissioned the development of a vibrational apparatus which, when used expose the patient to pulsate with vibrations – this was done using a variety of devices.

This hypothetical benefit of vibrations was maintained by Charcot as noticed an amelioration of symptoms among PD patients during long bouts of transport (e.g., carriage rides, trains), which appeared to contain a rhythmically vibrating component.[2]

Despite Charcot's stance against then present-day pharmacological agents, several neurologists continued experimenting with agents during the management of PD among their patients.[2] W.R. Gowers, a British neurologist noted that limited quantities of arsenic, cannabis, morphia and conium were effective agents in the temporary reduction of tremors.[6] He also noted a relationship between mental and physical strain between PD symptoms stating;

"life should be quiet and regular, freed, as far as may be, from care and work.". [6]

Gowers' recommendation on mental strain, in-part, continues to be clinically relevant today.[1]

The 20th century observed the greatest advent towards the management of PD. However, the discoveries representing progress were accompanied with a large trail of unsuccessful attempts. Surgical attempts, for example, targeted several regions of the brain in efforts to treat and prevent tremors among PD patients. The role of surgery grew surged towards the early and mid 1900s.[2] However, high mortality rates, lack-of-follow-up care, and worries for incomplete reporting by surgeon soon reduced surgical procedures for a newer pharmacological intervention, Levodopa.[7]

The discovery of dopamine as a key neurochemical player in the control of movement occurred in the 1950s, dopamine-loss was therefore naturally investigated alongside PD. A loss of dopaminergic neurons in the basal ganglia, a cluster of neurons primarily responsible for motor control/movement was identified as the key contributor towards the primary clinical features of PD.[1,7] In the 1960s, laboratory-developed levodopa, the precursor to dopamine, began trials among human patients. After a continual course of intravenous levodopa, significant changes in PD associated were reported:

"bed-ridden patients who were unable to sit up, patients who could not stand up when seated, and patients who when standing could not start walking performed all these activities with ease after L-dopa [levodopa]. They walked around with normal associated movements, and they could even run and jump. The voiceless, aphonic speech, blurred by pallilalia and unclear articulation, became forceful and clear as in a normal person." [8].

After the advent of levodopa, a largely pharmacological basis of levodopa-related treatments continues to be administered as the most prominent manner in addressing PD patients alongside manual therapy interventions aimed at improving the motor capabilities of patients.[2]

Epidemiology

PD is a multi-faceted illness which has climbed the ranks among neurodegenerative disorders to become the second most common, only behind Alzheimer's disease.[8] More recently, it has displayed the greatest increase in prevalence and disability among neurological disorders. Similarly, it has also grown to become a leading contributor to disability. Over the last few decades, for an abundance of reasons PD has become prevalent globally among aging populations and thus placing an increased burden among healthcare systems, medical professionals and caregivers alike. Statistics based on PD data between 1990-2019 have revealed 150% + increases in PD incidence and prevalence respectively.[10]

Compared to female patients, male patients had a larger incidence and prevalence number although both male and female patients have displayed alarming increases over time.[10] PD has been overwhelmingly common among older adults.[8] The largest increasing percentage occurred among those over 65 years.[10] Regionally, increases in incidence vary between region and sociodemographic factors. High-income North America incurred a drastic 296% incident increase compared to 27.5% within Eastern Europe. Despite the vast differences, the overall age-standardized incidence rate appeared increased among 18 of the 21 geographic regions which were accounted for in the most recent global-scale study.[10] Considering PD's chronicity and disability-inducing progression, the global years lived with disability (YLD) has also increased significantly (154.7%) over the 30-year span indicating an increase in experienced disability endured among PD patients.[8,10]

The tremendous increases in PD prevalence and incidence have been associated with several factors, markedly population growth and aging. Global growth in life expectancy is thought to work alongside lifestyle changes (i.e., presence/absence of risk behaviours),[11] genetic predisposition[12] and environmental pollution to varyingly contribute to the increased burden of PD.[13] Such factors may also explain the disparity between prevalence, incidence among males and females. Occupational factors and unhealthy behaviors (such as smoking, drinking, etc.) may facilitate poorer outcomes.[13] Analysis of the socio-demographic index also displayed significant trends attached to geographic/demographic-based regions. PD prevalence was higher in regions that had higher income, larger amount of population aging and decreased fertility rates.[13] As a result, the most pronounced increases of PD were seen among developed countries such as United States, Norway, and Germany.[13] Advances in disease management and treatment of PD has elucidated advantages despite increase in disease burden. Improved methods of detection, diagnosis and management has expected to increase the life expectancy of PD patients. However, it must be noted that access to sustainable, frequent, and high-quality care is far from equal globally. Thus, increases in PD-life-expectancy although estimated to grow may not manifest equally. [8,10,13]

Diagnosis

PD is the most common type of Parkinsonism, representing larger group neurological disorders displaying motor symptoms of rigidity, slowness and tremors. Clinically speaking, PD causes movement-related (motor) symptoms as well as non-movement related (non motor) symptoms. Motor symptoms usually consist of; tremor (involuntary rhythmic movement of one or part of the body, usually occurring within a person limb[s]), stiffness, slowness, and imbalance, postural instability. Conversely, non motor symptoms consist of; olfactory loss (loss or decreased sense of smell), sleep dysfunction, psychiatric issues (apathy, anxiety, depression, psychosis), cognitive impairments, in addition to a series of autonomic symptoms. The diagnosis of PD is typically based on the motor symptoms. However non motor symptoms develop gradually, often much before the manifestation of motor symptoms.[14] For this reason, PD patients are said to undergo a "prodromal phase" where several non motor symptoms develop. Research has determined that many patients often ignore or undisclosed these symptoms unless specifically queried.[14]

The occurrence of prodromal non motor symptoms are often associated with dysfunction and eventually pathology within select brain tissue. Neuropathology characterized by the death of dopaminergic neurons in the substantia nigra is a key element of PD pathophysiology.[14] However, the phasic development of PD has been attached to the BRAAK hypothesis[15] which postulates the genesis of PD in damage to the medulla and olfactory bulb. This is consistent with the non motor symptoms of sleep dysfunction and decreased smell. The disease then appears to advance to midbrain and forebrain structures (i.e. substantia nigra) which are responsible for the motor symptoms synonymous with PD.[14] Further neuropathological is detrimental to cerebral cortices which often cause greater cognitive impairment and hallucinations. The detection and diagnosis of PD typically occurs with the manifestation of motor symptoms.

The assessment is primarily based on a physical examination alongside an investigation of the symptoms of the patients. Family history is also discussed. Clinical criteria of PD requires the patient has parkinsonism (i.e bradykinesia, rigidity and/or tremor). A physical examination may include; decreased arm swing (when walking) , hypophonia, micrographia, short step length (when walking). Investigations on the patient's medical history may include a larger list of applicable non motor/motor symptoms including: slowness, soft voice, decreased facial expression, depression and/ or anxiety. In complex cases, the confirmation of a PD may occur using medical imaging in the form of a Dopamine transporter single-photon emission computed tomography (DaT SPECT). DaT SPECT can also be used to determine the presence of PD in cases where a direct evaluation of symptoms and patient history proves inconclusive. This form of imaging detects neuronal dysfunction relative to dopaminergic neurons.[16] Recent evidence has provided strong evidence of heterogeneity among PD symptoms and the manifestation of pathology among patients. For this reason, PD may be grouped in three groups based on motor/non motor symptoms; mild motor predominate, intermediate, diffuse malignant.[17] Mild motor predominate refers to a younger age of onset (younger older adulthood) with mild symptoms, slow disease progression and stronger response to medication. Intermediate group refers to faster disease progression, moderate-to-good response and slight older age of onset. Finally, diffuse malignant types display poor levodopa response, severe dopaminergic dysfunction, rapid progression, cognitive impairment, sleep dysfunction and orthostatic hypotension. [17]

Treatment

Given the progressiveness of PD combined with its chronicity, the treatments are targeted controlling motor/non motor symptoms rather than reversing the pathophysiology of disease. Thus, a combination of treatments used to manage symptoms while improve the extent of disability and quality of life of patients.[17]

Motor symptoms are primarily treated using dopamine-based agents including varying preparations of levodopa, dopamine agonists and monoamine oxidase-B (MAO-B) inhibitors. However, selecting the appropriate treatment is multi-faceted considering the advantages of each agent combined with potential side effects. Levodopa appears to result in functional motor improvements.[18] However, increased dosage and continual usage appears to increase dyskinesia (involuntary erratic movements). On the other hand, dopamine agonists MAO-B inhibitors result in effectiveness managing milder motor symptoms and present lower dyskinesia risk. It must be noted that pharmacological agents for motor symptoms are often taken in combination to ensure symptom mitigation is upheld while reducing the risk for adverse reactions. [8,17,18]

In addition to pharmacological treatments, motor symptoms are also addressed using a variety of exercise-intervention including balance training, progressive resistance, gait training, strength training, aerobics among others.[19] Physiotherapy, massage, and occupational therapy have also demonstrated positive outcomes. As a result, interdisciplinary treatment using pharmacological along with movement-based treatments are vital in the management of motor symptoms.[19]

Persistent motor symptoms unresponsive to the prolonged exposure of the above-mentioned treatments can be addressed using more invasive treatments. Such treatments are highly specialized and thus require PD to adhere to strict guidelines.[17] Deep-brain stimulation (DBS), for example, surgical placement of leads in the subthalamic nucleus or the globus pallidus interna. These implanted leads, along with medication are used to treat severe motor symptoms. However, it must be noted that surgical procedures like DBS do present a consistent slightly increased risk of numbness, slurred speech and vision problems. [17]

Non motor symptoms demonstrate a wider range of maladies and are therefore managed using a wider range of pharmacological agents, primarily with neurotransmitters other than dopamine. Non motor symptoms are primarily addressed using drugs that would be used to address these symptoms among non-PD symptoms. For this reason, there is consistency between the prescribed agents to address non motor symptoms between PD and non-PD patients. This approach is fairly efficacious towards PD patients however results may vary.[17]

Future Directions

Pharmacological interventions approved for clinical use for PD have all been towards symptomatic relief rather than disease prevention. Resultantly, investigations on a variety of aspects including novel treatments, disease prevention strategies, patient monitoring solutions, diagnostic tools as well as disparities within the patient population have recognized and promoted.[21]

To begin with, research in the space of wearable technologies involving garments which can be worn by patients are currently being researched relevant to PD. These articles of clothing include a variety of sensors which can allow for the real time detection and cataloging of key biomarkers which can aid in diagnostic capabilities.[21,22] PD has been suspected to manifest differently in home settings compared to clinical interactions. As a result, remote measurements allow for accurate representation of patient-reported outcomes allowing for diagnostic capabilities, therefore leading to better treatment implementation.[22] In addition to better diagnostic methods, a large number of clinicians actively continue to investigate possibilities to slow and/or mitigate the progression of PD. These efforts, mostly pharmacological in nature, are underway in very early and limited stages.[23] Genetics mechanisms also continue to be explored to understand the onset of PD as well as predisposing characteristics. Factors such environmental agents and lifestyles also are explored retrospectively to elucidate non-modifiable and modifiable that are correlated with positive/negative PD outcomes.[24]

References

1. Parkinson's Disease and Its Management - PMC (nih.gov)

2. 10.1101/cshperspect.a008862

3. An Essay on the Shaking Palsy | The Journal of Neuropsychiatry and Clinical Neurosciences (psychiatryonline.org)

4. Lecons sur, les maladies du système nerveux - Jean Martin Charcot - Google Books

5. https://www.ncbi.nlm.nih.gov/pmc/articles/PMC3234454/#A008862C2

6. King's Collections : Online Exhibitions : Gowers on paralysis agitans (kingscollections.org)

7. 10.1212/wnl.50.6_suppl_6.s2

8. Poewe W, Seppi K, Tanner CM, Halliday GM, Brundin P, Volkmann J, et al. Parkinson disease. *Nat Rev Dis Primers.* (2017) 3:17013. doi: 10.1038/nrdp.2017.13

9. GBD Neurological Disorders Collaborator Group. Global, regional, and national burden of neurological disorders during 1990-2015: a systematic analysis for the Global Burden of Disease Study 2015. *Lancet Neurol.* (2017) 16:877–97. doi: 10.1016/S1474-4422(17)30299-5

10. https://doi.org/10.3389/fpubh.2021.776847

11. Doiron M, Dupre N, Langlois M, Provencher P. Smoking history is associated to cognitive impairment in Parkinson's disease. *Aging Ment Health.* (2017) 21:322–6. doi: 10.1080/13607863.2015.1090393

12. Alcalay RN, Kehoe C, Shorr E, Battista R, Hall A, Simuni T, et al. Genetic testing for Parkinson disease: current practice, knowledge, and attitudes among US and Canadian movement disorders specialists. *Genet Med.* (2020) 22:574–80. doi: 10.1038/s41436-019-0684-x

13. GBD Parkinson's Disease Collaborators. Global, regional, and national burden of Parkinson's disease, 1990-2016: a systematic analysis for the Global Burden of Disease Study 2016. *Lancet Neurol.* (2018) 17:939–53. doi: 10.1016/S1474-4422(18)30295-3

14. Diagnosis and Treatment of Parkinson Disease: A Review (uwo. ca)

15. Braak H, Del Tredici K, Rüb U, de Vos RA, Jansen Steur EN, Braak E. Staging of brain pathology related to sporadic Parkinson's disease. Neurobiol Aging. 2003;24(2):197-211. doi:10.1016/S0197-4580 (02)00065-9

16. Suwijn SR, van Boheemen CJ, de Haan RJ, Tissingh G, Booij J, de Bie RM. The diagnostic accuracy of dopamine transporter SPECT imaging to detect nigrostriatal cell loss in patients with Parkinson's disease or clinically uncertain parkinsonism: a systematic review. EJNMMI Res. 2015;5:12. doi:10.1186/s13550-015-0087-1

17. Fereshtehnejad SM, Zeighami Y, Dagher A, Postuma RB. Clinical criteria for subtyping Parkinson's disease: biomarkers and longitudinal progression. Brain. 2017;140(7):1959-1976. doi:10. 1093/brain/awx118

18. Turcano P, Mielke MM, Bower JH, et al. Levodopa-induced dyskinesia in Parkinson disease: a population-based cohort study. Neurology. 2018; 91(24):e2238-e2243. doi:10.1212/WNL. 0000000000006643

19. Mak MK, Wong-Yu IS, Shen X, Chung CL. Long-term effects of exercise and physical therapy in people with Parkinson disease. Nat Rev Neurol. 2017;13(11):689-703. doi:10.1038/nrneurol.2017.128

20. Factor SA, Bennett A, Hohler AD, Wang D, Miyasaki JM. Quality improvement in neurology: Parkinson disease update quality measurement set: executive summary. Neurology. 2016;86(24):2278

21. Silva de Lima AL, Hahn T, Evers LJW, et al. Feasibility of large-scale deployment of multiple wearable sensors in Parkinson's disease. PLoS One 2017; 12: e0189161.

22. Lin CH, Li CH, Yang KC, et al. Blood NfL: a biomarker for disease severity and progression in Parkinson disease. Neurology 2019; 93: e1104–11.

23. Brundin P, Wyse RK. The Linked Clinical Trials initiative (LCT) for Parkinson's disease. Eur J Neurosci 2019; 49: 307–15.

24. Dorsey ER, Sherer T, Okun MS, Bloem BR. The emerging evidence of the Parkinson pandemic. J Parkinsons Dis 2018; 8: S3–8

www.ingramcontent.com/pod-product-compliance
Lightning Source LLC
Chambersburg PA
CBHW031814190326

41518CB00006B/340